Table of Contents

Kidney cancer develops when cells in your kidneys change and grow out of control. People with kidney cancer may notice flank pain, high blood pressure, blood in their pee and other symptoms. Kidney cancer treatments include surgery, chemotherapy and radiation therapy. As with all cancers, early detection is key for successful treatment. The kidneys are a pair of bean-shaped organs, each about the size of a fist. They are attached to the upper back wall of the abdomen and protected by the lower rib cage. One kidney is just to the left and the other just to the right of the backbone. The upper and lower portions of each kidney are sometimes called the superior pole and inferior pole. A small organ called an adrenal gland sits on top of each kidney. Each kidney and adrenal gland is surrounded by fat and a thin, fibrous layer known as Gerota's fascia. The kidneys' main job is to remove excess water, salt, and waste products from blood coming in from the renal arteries. These substances become urine. Urine collects in the center of each kidney in an area called the renal pelvis and then leaves the kidneys through long slender tubes called ureters. The ureters lead to the bladder, where the urine is stored until you urinate.

The kidneys also have other jobs

• They help control blood pressure by making a hormone called renin.

• They help make sure the body has enough red blood cells by making a hormone called erythropoietin. This hormone tells the bone marrow to make more red blood cells.

• Our kidneys are important, but we can function with only one kidney. Many people in the United States are living normal, healthy lives with just one kidney.

Some people do not have working kidneys at all, and survive with the help of a medical procedure called dialysis. The most common form of dialysis uses a specially designed machine that filters blood much like a real kidney would.

Kidney cancer is the abnormal growth of cells in your kidney tissue. In time, these cells form a mass called a tumor. Cancer begins when something triggers a change in the cells, and they divide out of control. A cancerous or malignant tumor can spread to other tissues and vital organs. When this happens, it's called metastasis.

Types of kidney cancer

Renal cell carcinoma

Renal cell carcinoma (RCC), also known as renal cell cancer or renal cell adenocarcinoma, is the most common type of kidney cancer. About 9 out of 10 kidney cancers are renal cell carcinomas.

Although RCC usually grows as a single tumor within a kidney, sometimes there are 2 or more tumors in one kidney or even tumors in both kidneys at the same time.

There are several subtypes of RCC, based mainly on how the cancer cells look in the lab. Knowing the subtype of RCC can be a factor in deciding treatment and can also help your doctor determine if your cancer might be caused by an inherited genetic syndrome. See Risk Factors for Kidney Cancer for more information about inherited kidney cancer syndromes.

Clear cell renal cell carcinoma

This is the most common form of renal cell carcinoma. About 7 out of 10 people with RCC have this kind of cancer. When seen in the lab, the cells that make up clear cell RCC look very pale or clear.

Non-clear cell renal cell carcinomas

Papillary renal cell carcinoma: This is the second most common subtype – about 1 in 10 RCCs are of this type. These cancers form little finger-like projections (called papillae) in some, if not most, of the tumor. Some doctors call these cancers chromophilic because the cells take in certain dyes and look pink when looked at under the microscope.

Chromophobe renal cell carcinoma: This subtype accounts for about 5% (5 cases in 100) of RCCs. The cells of these cancers are also pale, like the clear cells, but are much larger and have certain other features that can be recognized when looked at very closely.

Rare types of renal cell carcinoma: These subtypes are very rare, each making up less than 1% of RCCs:

• Collecting duct RCC

• Multilocular cystic RCC

• Medullary carcinoma

• Mucinous tubular and spindle cell carcinoma

• Neuroblastoma-associated RCC

Unclassified renal cell carcinoma: Rarely, renal cell cancers are labeled as unclassified because the way they look doesn't fit into any of the other categories or because there is more than one type of cancer cell present.

Other types of kidney cancers

Other types of kidney cancers include transitional cell carcinomas, Wilms tumors, and renal sarcomas.

Transitional cell carcinoma: Of every 100 cancers in the kidney, about 5 to 10 are transitional cell carcinomas (TCCs), also known as urothelial carcinomas.

Transitional cell carcinomas don't start in the kidney itself, but in the lining of the renal pelvis (where the ureters meet the kidneys). This lining is made up of cells called transitional cells that look like the cells that line the ureters and bladder. Cancers that develop from these cells look like other urothelial carcinomas, such as bladder cancer, when looked at closely in the lab. Like bladder cancer, these cancers are often linked to cigarette smoking and being exposed to certain cancer-causing chemicals in the workplace.

People with TCC often have the same signs and symptoms as people with renal cell cancer − blood in the urine and, sometimes, back pain.

Wilms tumor (nephroblastoma): Wilms tumors almost always occur in children. This type of cancer is very rare among adults.

Renal sarcoma: Renal sarcomas are a rare type of kidney cancer that begin in the blood vessels or connective tissue of the kidney. They make up less than 1% of all kidney cancers.

Sarcomas are discussed in more detail in Sarcoma- Adult Soft Tissue Cancer.

Benign (non-cancerous) kidney tumors

Some kidney tumors are benign (non-cancer). This means they do not metastasize (spread) to other parts of the body, although they can still grow and cause problems.

Benign kidney tumors can be treated by removing or destroying them, using many of the same treatments that are also used for kidney cancers, such as surgery or radiofrequency ablation. The choice of treatment depends on many factors, such as the size of the tumor and if it is causing any symptoms, the number of tumors, whether tumors are in both kidneys, and the person's general health.

Angiomyolipoma: Angiomyolipomas are the most common benign kidney tumor. They are seen more often in women. They can develop sporadically or in people with tuberous sclerosis, a genetic condition that also affects the heart, eyes, brain, lungs, and skin.

These tumors are made up of different types of connective tissues (blood vessels, smooth muscles, and fat). If they aren't causing any symptoms, they can often just be watched closely. If they start causing problems (like pain or bleeding), they may need to be treated.

Oncocytoma: Oncocytomas are benign kidney tumors that are not common and can sometimes grow quite large. They are seen more often in men and do not normally spread to other organs, so surgery often cures them.

How common is kidney cancer

Kidney cancer represents about 3.7% of all cancers in the United States. Each year, more than 62,000 Americans are diagnosed with kidney cancer. The risk of kidney cancer increases with age.

What are the signs of kidney cancer?

Kidney cancer may not produce any noticeable symptoms in its early stages. But as the tumor grows, symptoms may begin to appear. For that reason, kidney cancer often isn't diagnosed until it has begun to spread.

Kidney cancer symptoms may include:

• Blood in your pee (hematuria).

• A lump or mass in your kidney area.

• Flank pain.

• Tiredness.

• A general sense of not feeling well.

• Loss of appetite.

• Weight loss.

• Low-grade fever.

• Bone pain.

• High blood pressure.

• Anemia.

• High calcium.

What is the primary cause of kidney cancer

The exact cause of kidney cancer isn't known, but there are certain risk factors that may increase your chances of getting the disease. These include:

• Smoking: People who smoke are at greater risk for kidney cancer. In addition, the longer a person smokes, the higher the risk.

• Obesity: Obesity is a risk factor for kidney cancer. In general, the more overweight a person is, the higher the risk.

• High blood pressure: Also called hypertension, high blood pressure has been linked to an increased risk of kidney cancer.

• Family history: People who have family members with kidney cancer may have an increased risk of developing cancer themselves.

• Radiation therapy: Women who have been treated with radiation for cancer of their reproductive organs may have a slightly increased risk of developing kidney cancer.

• Gene changes (mutations): Genes contain instructions for a cell's function. Changes in certain genes can increase the risk of developing kidney cancer.

• Long-term dialysis treatment: Dialysis is the process of cleaning your blood by passing it through a special machine. Dialysis is used when a person's kidneys aren't functioning properly.

• Tuberous sclerosis complex: Tuberous sclerosis is a disease that causes seizures and intellectual disabilities, as well as the formation of tumors in many different organs.

• Von Hippel-Lindau disease (VHL): People with this inherited disorder are at greater risk for developing kidney cancer. This disorder causes noncancerous tumors in your blood vessels, typically in your eyes and brain.

It depends. Some kidney tumors are benign (noncancerous). These tumors are generally smaller than cancerous tumors and don't spread to other parts of your body. Surgical removal is the most common treatment for noncancerous kidney tumors. Whether your kidney tumor is cancerous or noncancerous, you should move forward with treatment as soon as possible to avoid complications.

How is kidney cancer diagnosed

If you have kidney cancer symptoms, your healthcare provider will perform a complete medical history and physical exam. They also may order certain tests that can help in diagnosing and assessing cancer. These tests may include:

Urinalysis: A sample of your urine (pee) is tested to see if it contains blood. Even very small traces of blood, invisible to the naked eye, can be detected in tests of urine samples.

Blood tests: These tests count the number of each of the different kinds of blood cells, as well as look at different electrolytes in your body. A blood test can show if there are too few red blood cells (anemia), or if your kidney function is impaired (by looking at the creatinine).

CT scan: This is a special X-ray that uses a computer to create a series of images, or slices, of the inside of your body. This test is often done with intravenous contrast (dye). People with impaired kidney function may not be able to receive the dye.

Magnetic resonance imaging (MRI): This is a test that produces images of the inside of your body using a large magnet, radio waves and a computer.

Ultrasound: This test uses high-frequency sound waves that are transmitted through body tissues to create images that are displayed on a monitor. This test is helpful in detecting tumors, which have a different density from healthy tissues.

Renal mass biopsy: During this procedure, a thin needle is inserted into the tumor, and a small sample of your tissue is removed (biopsy). A pathologist will look at the tissue under a microscope to see if there are any cancer cells. Because biopsies for kidney cancer aren't always completely reliable, your healthcare provider may or may not recommend this test.

Most cancers are grouped by stage, a description of cancer that aids in planning treatment. The stage of a cancer is based on:

• The location and size of the tumor.

• The extent to which your lymph nodes are affected.

• The degree to which the cancer spread, if at all, to other tissue and organs.

Your healthcare provider uses information from various tests, including CT, MRI and biopsy, to determine the stage of cancer.

Stage I: The tumor is 7 centimeters (cm) across or smaller and is only in your kidney. It hasn't spread to lymph nodes or other tissue. (Lymph nodes are small "filters" that trap germs and cancer cells and store infection-fighting cells.).

Stage II: The tumor is larger than 7 cm across but is still only in your kidney. It hasn't spread to lymph nodes or other tissue.

Stage III: The tumor has spread to your major blood vessels — your renal vein and inferior vena cava — or into the tissue surrounding your kidney or to nearby lymph nodes.

Stage IV: The tumor has spread outside of your kidney to your adrenal gland (the small gland that sits on top of your kidney), or to distant lymph nodes or other organs.

Tumors are also graded, which is a way of rating a tumor based on how abnormal its cells look. Tumor grading can also tell your healthcare provider how fast the tumor is likely to grow. Tumors whose cells don't look like normal cells and divide rapidly are called high-grade tumors. High-grade tumors tend to grow and spread more quickly than low-grade tumors.

Management And Treatment

How is kidney cancer treated?

Kidney cancer treatment depends on the stage and grade of the tumor, as well as your age and overall health. Options include surgery, ablation, radiation therapy, targeted drug therapy, immunotherapy and sometimes chemotherapy.

Surgery

Surgery is the treatment of choice for most stages of kidney cancer. Several surgical options may be considered, including:

• Partial nephrectomy: Your surgeon removes the part of your kidney that contains the tumor.

• Radical nephrectomy: Your surgeon removes your entire kidney and some of the tissue around it. They may also remove some lymph nodes in the area. When one kidney is removed, the remaining kidney is usually able to perform the work of both kidneys.

Ablation

Sometimes, heat and cold can destroy cancer cells. People who aren't candidates for surgery may benefit from cryoablation or radiofrequency ablation.

Cryoablation: During this procedure, your healthcare provider inserts a needle through your skin and into the kidney tumor. The cancer cells are then frozen with cold gas.

Radiofrequency ablation: Your healthcare provider inserts a needle through your skin and into the kidney tumor. Next, an electrical current is passed through the cancer cells to destroy them.

Radiation therapy

Your healthcare provider may recommend radiation therapy if you only have one kidney or if you're not eligible for surgery. Radiation therapy is most often used for easing kidney cancer symptoms, such as pain.

Targeted drug therapy

Targeted drug therapy blocks certain characteristics that help cancer cells thrive. For example, these drugs can stop the growth of new blood vessels or proteins that feed cancer.

Targeted drug therapy is often used when surgery isn't an option. In some cases, these medications may be given after surgery to reduce the risk of cancer coming back.

Immunotherapy

Immunotherapy uses certain medications to boost your own immune system. In turn, this helps your body recognize and destroy cancer cells more effectively. Immunotherapy may be given as a standalone treatment or along with surgery.

Chemotherapy

Chemotherapy isn't a standard treatment for kidney cancer. But it can be helpful in some cases — usually only after trying immunotherapy and targeted drug therapy. Chemotherapy medications are taken by mouth or given through a vein (intravenously) and are generally well tolerated.

What Causes Kidney Masses?

There is no known cause for developing a kidney mass. But there are a number of things that can increase your risk for kidney tumors such as:

• Smoking

• Obesity, poor diet

• High blood pressure

• Being on kidney dialysis

• Workplace exposure to chlorinated chemicals

• Heredity, which accounts for about 4-6% of kidney cancer cases

What are the Symptoms of a Kidney Mass?

Most kidney masses have no symptoms in the early stages. If there are symptoms, they will most likely be:

• Hematuria (blood in urine)

• Flank pain between the ribs and hips

• Low back pain on one side (not caused by injury) that does not go away

• Loss of appetite

• Weight loss not caused by dieting

• Fever that is not caused by an infection and does not go away

• Anemia (low red blood cell count)

What to eat

Eating a nutritious, balanced diet is a good idea for everyone — but especially those who are living with kidney cancer. While your nutritional needs may depend on what type of treatment you're on and the stage of your cancer, there are a few foods you should make an effort to include in all of your meals, if possible:

Fruits and vegetables

Fruits and vegetables are high in fiber and a good source of many essential vitamins and minerals. They can also help to reduce cholesterol levels and can help manage your blood sugar. Fiber-rich vegetables, such as beans and peas, are also healthful.

You should aim to have 4 servings of fruit and 5 servings of vegetables from a variety of sources every day.

A few sample servings are:

• 1 medium apple

• 6 baby carrots

• 16 grapes

• half of a medium potato

• 1 cup raw leafy greens

• Whole grains

• Whole wheat bread, wild rice, and whole wheat pasta are excellent sources of energy. They're also rich in fiber, iron, and B vitamins.

Certain whole grains, like some whole-grain breads and bran products, can be high in phosphorus. While this common mineral shouldn't cause an issue for people with healthy kidneys, consuming too much when your kidneys aren't functioning properly may cause some health problems. This is because the kidneys help to balance the amount of phosphorus in your body.

Phosphorus is in a lot of foods, and small amounts of it should still be OK even if you're living with kidney cancer. However, your doctor's advice about your personal phosphorus intake should always take priority over general guidelines.

Proteins

Proteins are a necessary part of everyone's diet, as they help to build and maintain muscle mass. But too much protein for someone with kidney cancer may cause a buildup of food-derived waste in the bloodstream. This may cause symptoms like fatigue, nausea, and headache. Speak with a doctor or a registered dietitian about the right amount and best types of protein to include in your diet.

Several foods can increase your risk of kidney-related complications. If it's not possible to avoid these foods or habits, try to limit your intake when possible.

Foods that are high in salt

Too much salt can disrupt the fluid balance in your body and lead to high blood pressure. This can exacerbate the symptoms of reduced kidney function.

Processed foods are typically high in sodium, so when possible, try to eat less of:

• Fast food

• Salty snacks (like potato chips)

• Processed deli meats (like salami)

Whenever possible, use herbs and spices for flavoring instead of salt. However, if you're using unconventional herbs, check with your doctor.

Foods high in phosphorus

Again, phosphorusis a natural mineral that helps your body in a variety of ways, including contributing to bone strength. But in people with reduced kidney function due to cancer, too much phosphorus can actually weaken your bones, as well as cause other side effects.

If your doctor is concerned about your phosphorus intake, they may recommend you reduce the amount of phosphorus-rich foods you consume, such as:

• Cocoa

• Beans

• Processed bran cereals

• Certain dairy products

• Oysters

Too much water

Overhydrating may also create problems for people with kidney cancer. Having reduced kidney function can compromise your urine production and cause your body to retain too much fluid. It's important for everyone to drink plenty of water, but make an effort to monitor your intake of fluids so you're not consuming an excessive amount.

Highly processed foods and beverages

A 2018 prospective study found a 10 percent increase in cancer risk for people who eat ultra-processed foods. Mortality risk has been associated with lower levels of diet quality. Red and processed meats have corresponded with lower dietary quality.

Try to limit highly processed foods and beverages, such as:

• Packaged bread and snacks

• Sodas and sweetened drinks

• Meat preserved with nitrates

• Instant noodles and soups

• Frozen or shelf-stable ready meals

• Alcohol

Beer, wine, and liquor could interact with the cancer drugs you take. There is also some limited evidence that drinking alcohol may increase the risk of recurrence and mortality for existing cancer.

How You Should Eat

The side effects of your cancer treatment will have a lot to do with your diet. Here are some problems you may face, along with potential solutions.

Poor appetite Cancer treatment can wipe out your appetite, but you still need to eat. To make sure you get the nutrition you need, try to:

• Have five or six small meals during the day instead of three large ones.

• Keep small snacks handy for when you feel like eating.

• Eat as much as you can when your appetite is strongest, usually early in the morning.

• Focus on the foods you can eat without difficulty, even if there are only a couple of them.

• Drink a shake or a smoothie if a full meal is unappealing.

Nausea Lots of different things can nauseate you during kidney cancer treatment. To avoid it, you might:

• Choose bland foods, such as white toast, plain yogurt, and clear broth, and avoid spicy, sour, or acidic foods.

• Eat foods that are room temperature, rather than cold or hot.

• Limit the number of beverages you consume with meals and instead get your fluids in between meals — and take smaller sips.

• Make sure you don't skip meals and snacks. An empty stomach is more likely to make you feel nauseous.

• Avoid your most loved foods while you are nauseated. Although it may seem counterintuitive, if you try to eat your favorite foods when you are sick, you may develop an aversion to them.

Weakness Kidney cancer treatment can rob you of energy. To make sure you eat enough despite fatigue and weakness, you should:

• Stock up on foods that are easily prepared, such as canned soups — your doctor may prefer that you purchase low-sodium varieties — frozen dinners, and precooked meals.

• Cook meals ahead of time, when you're feeling well, and freeze them for later.

• Ask friends, prior to treatment, to help you shop and cook when you're not feeling well later on.

• Plan for foods that come in thick liquid (milkshakes) or semisolid (mashed potatoes) form for when you are too weak to chew properly.

• Get groceries delivered to your home if going shopping is not feasible.

Mouth sores It's common for kidney cancer patients who are being treated with targeted drugs and immunotherapy to experience inflammation, irritation, and ulceration of the mouth, esophagus, and other parts of the gastrointestinal tract. If you're having trouble eating due to these issues, Prest suggests the following:

• Choose nutrient-dense, soft, moist, easy-to-chew foods.

• Avoid acidic foods, alcohol, and spicy foods.

• Choose foods that are not too cold or too hot.

• Practice good oral hygiene with a soft toothbrush.

Talk to your doctor about using pain meds or a topical analgesic mouth rinse before meals.

Increased risk of infection Certain cancer treatments, such as radiation therapy, or even the cancer itself can ravage the immune system and leave you open to infection, according to the ACS. "Pay attention to the four principles of food safety: Clean, separate, cook, and chill," Prest says. You — or the person preparing your meals — should:

• Thoroughly wash and scrub fruits and vegetables.

• Wash your hands, clean knives, and scrub down countertops before and after you prepare food, especially raw meat.

• Keep cooked and raw foods separate to avoid cross-contamination.

• Use a different cutting board and utensils for raw and cooked foods.

• Fully cook meats, poultry, and eggs. Meat should have no pink; eggs should not be runny.

• Store leftovers in the refrigerator immediately after eating.

• Drink only pasteurized milk or fruit juice.

• Avoid uncooked shellfish or raw fish.

• Pass on any foods that show signs of mold, including moldy cheeses such as blue cheese.

• Pay attention to freshness dates and don't eat expired foods.

Other tips to keep in mind:

• If you're experiencing vomiting or diarrhea, be sure to sip small amounts of water or broth (per your doctor's recommendations) throughout the day to replenish lost fluid.

• Kidney cancer treatments such as immunotherapy medications and targeted therapy drugs can increase your risk of high blood pressure and cholesterol. By working with your dietitian, you can make a healthy eating plan that can keep this risk in mind and still give you the calories and nutrition you need.

Tips for how to eat during treatment

While a varied, nutrient-dense diet is one of the best ways to care for yourself, going through cancer treatment can have varying effects on your body and your appetite.

Poor appetite

It's common to lose weight during treatment for many types of cancer, including kidney cancer. You may find that your taste for certain foods changes. Things that used to appeal to you may no longer be appetizing and may even make you feel nauseous.

But you can use trial and error to find a few go-to foods that don't make you feel sick.

Even if you're not feeling particularly hungry, try your best to eat regular meals so that your energy levels remain consistent throughout the day. If you have trouble eating full-sized portions, it may help to break up your meals into five or six smaller servings instead of the typical two or three big ones.

Eat your biggest meal when you're hungriest — no matter what time of day it is.

Nutrition bars and smoothies may be good options to get extra calories in if your appetite isn't what it used to be. Talk with your doctor or a registered dietitian about the healthiest options.

Weakness

It's common to deal with energy changes while going through cancer treatment. You may have less energy than normal and may even deal with weakness and fatigue.

Talk with your doctor, dietitian, spouse, or caregiver about meal delivery options. There's a variety of these available, and many of them have nutrition information front and center. They can help make meal prep a snap, as well as help you eat your desired amount of calories.

There are certain foods that may be especially helpful for maintaining energy, as well as being easy to prepare. A few of them include:

• Fruits

• Nuts and nut butters

• Vegetables with healthier dips like hummus

• Sandwhiches with leaner protein (turkey, chicken, peanut butter)

• Cheese

• Hardboiled eggs

• Whole grain cereals

• Low sugar granola bars

• Yogurt

• Smoothies

Other side effects

Cancer treatment can weaken your immune system and make you more susceptible to infection. Because of this, you may want to take these precautions while preparing and storing your meals:

• Wash produce thoroughly.

• Use separate cutting boards for meats and vegetables.

• Make sure all foods like meat, poultry, and eggs are well cooked.

• Avoid drinking unpasteurized milk or juice.

• Be vary careful around raw foods like sushi, shellfish, and vegetable sprouts.

• Toss anything that looks slimy or moldy, especially produce.

You may deal with mouth sores or swallowing issues while going through certain types of treatment. If this is the case, there are some methods that may help you maintain your daily caloric and nutrient goals:

• Use a soft toothbrush to take care of your dental health.

• Talk with your doctor about steroids or anti-inflammatory drugs to help manage the pain and symptoms.

• Avoid spicy foods.

• Limit acidic juices and fruits like lemons and orange juice.

• Focus on small meals and foods that are easy to chew, like yogurt, smoothies, and pureed soups.

Recipes

Avocado deviled eggs

Ingredients

• 6 eggs, hard boiled

• 1 ripe avocado, peeled and pitted

• 1 1/2 teaspoons lime juice

• 3 tablespoons light mayonnaise

• 1 teaspoon chopped parsley

• 2 teaspoons ground cayenne pepper

• 2 cloves fresh garlic, minced

Directions

• Cut eggs lengthwise and remove yolks. Set aside half the yolks in bowl and discard the others.

• In a medium bowl combine egg yolks, avocado, lime juice, mayonnaise, half of the parsley, cayenne pepper and garlic. Spoon mixture into egg whites and garnish with other half of chopped parsley.

Baba ghanoush

Ingredients

• 1 bulb garlic (about 8 cloves)

• 2 eggplants, sliced lengthwise, skin removed

• 1 red bell pepper, halved and seeded

• Juice of 1 lemon (about 4 tablespoons)

• 1 tablespoon chopped fresh basil

• 1 tablespoon olive oil

• 1 teaspoon black pepper or to taste

• 2 rounds of whole-wheat pita or other flatbread

Directions

• Spray cold grill with cooking spray. Heat one side of the grill to high. (Or move coals to one side of the grill.)

• Slice top off garlic bulb, wrap in foil and place on cooler part of grill. Roast for 20 to 30 minutes. On hot part of grill, place eggplant slices and bell pepper. Grill for 2 to 3 minutes on each side.

• Squeeze roasted garlic out of bulb and place in food processor. Add grilled eggplant and red bell pepper. Add lemon juice, basil, olive oil and pepper. Pulse until smooth. Place dip in serving bowl.

• Warm bread on grill for a few seconds on each side. Serve with dip.

Ingredients

• 20 crimini mushrooms, washed and stems removed

Topping:

• 1 1/2 cups panko breadcrumbs

• 1/4 cup melted butter

• 3 tablespoons chopped fresh parsley

Filling:

• 2 cups fresh basil leaves

• 1/4 cup fresh Parmesan cheese

• 2 tablespoons pumpkin seeds

• 1 tablespoon olive oil

• 1 tablespoon fresh garlic

• 2 teaspoons lemon juice

• 1/2 teaspoon kosher salt

Directions

• Heat the oven to 350 F. Line the mushroom caps upside down on a baking sheet.

• To prepare the topping, in a small bowl, combine the panko, butter and parsley; set aside.

• To prepare the filling, place the basil, cheese, pumpkin seeds, oil, garlic, lemon juice and salt in a food processor. Process until evenly mixed.

• Generously stuff the mushroom caps with the basil pesto filling. Sprinkle each mushroom with about 1 teaspoon of panko topping. Gently pat down the topping. Bake for 10 to 15 minutes or until golden brown.

Fruit salsa and sweet chips

Ingredients

For tortilla crisps:

• 8 whole-wheat fat-free tortillas

• Cooking spray

• 1 tablespoon sugar

• 1/2 tablespoon cinnamon

For fruit salsa:

• 3 cups diced fresh fruit, such as apples, oranges, kiwi, strawberries, grapes or other fresh fruit

• 2 tablespoons sugar-free jam, any flavor

• 1 tablespoon honey or agave nectar

• 2 tablespoons orange juice

Directions

• Heat the oven to 350 F. Cut each tortilla into 8 wedges. Lay pieces on two baking sheets. Make sure they aren't overlapping. Spray the tortilla pieces with cooking spray.

• In a small bowl, combine sugar and cinnamon. Sprinkle evenly over the tortilla wedges. Bake for 10 to 12 minutes or until the pieces are crisp. Place on a cooling rack and let cool.

• Cut the fruit into cubes. Gently mix the fruit together in a mixing bowl. In another bowl, whisk together jam, honey and orange juice. Pour this over the diced fruit. Mix gently. Cover the bowl with plastic wrap and refrigerate for 2 to 3 hours.

• Serve as a dip or topping for the cinnamon tortilla chips.

Ingredients

For the marinade

• 2 tablespoons dark honey

• 1 tablespoon olive oil

• 1 tablespoon fresh lime juice

• 1 teaspoon ground cinnamon

• 1/4 teaspoon ground cloves

• 1 firm, ripe pineapple

• 8 wooden skewers, soaked in water for 30 minutes, or metal skewers

• 1 tablespoon dark rum (optional)

• 1 tablespoon grated lime zest

Directions

• Prepare a hot fire in a charcoal grill or heat a gas grill or broiler. Away from the heat source, lightly coat the grill rack or broiler pan with cooking spray. Position the cooking rack 4 to 6 inches from the heat source.

• To make the marinade, in a small bowl, combine the honey, olive oil, lime juice, cinnamon and cloves and whisk to blend. Set aside.

• Cut off the crown of leaves and the base of the pineapple. Stand the pineapple upright and, using a large, sharp knife, pare off the skin, cutting downward just below the surface in long, vertical strips and leaving the small brown "eyes" on the fruit.

• Lay the pineapple on its side. Aligning the knife blade with the diagonal rows of eyes, cut a shallow furrow, following a spiral pattern around the pineapple, to remove all the eyes.

• Stand the peeled pineapple upright and cut it in half lengthwise. Place each pineapple half cut-side down and cut it lengthwise into four long wedges. Slice away the core. Cut each wedge crosswise into three pieces. Thread the three pineapple pieces onto each skewer.

• Lightly brush the pineapple with the marinade. Grill or broil, turning once and basting once or twice with the remaining marinade, until tender and golden, about 5 minutes on each side.

• Remove the pineapple from the skewers and place on a platter or individual serving plates. Brush with the rum, if using, and sprinkle with the lime zest. Serve hot or warm.

Hummus

Ingredients

• 2 cans (16 ounces each) reduced-sodium chickpeas, rinsed and drained except for 1/4 cup liquid

• 1 tablespoon extra-virgin olive oil

• 1/4 cup lemon juice

• 2 garlic cloves, minced

• 1/4 teaspoon cracked black pepper

• 1/4 teaspoon paprika

• 3 tablespoons tahini (sesame paste)*

• 2 tablespoons chopped Italian flat-leaf parsley

*Note: If you need to follow a gluten-free diet, check the label to make sure the brand of tahini is gluten-free.

Directions

• Using a blender or food processor, puree the chickpeas. Add the olive oil, lemon juice, garlic, pepper, paprika, tahini and parsley. Blend well.

• Add the reserved liquid, 1 tablespoon at a time, until the mixture has the consistency of a thick spread.

• Serve immediately or cover and refrigerate until ready to serve.

Roasted red pepper hummus

Ingredients

• 2 cups canned chickpeas, rinsed and drained

• 1 cup roasted red bell pepper, slices, seeded

• 2 tablespoons white sesame seeds

• 1 tablespoon lemon juice

• 1 tablespoon olive oil

• 1 1/4 teaspoons cumin

• 1 teaspoon onion powder

• 1 teaspoon garlic powder

• 1 teaspoon kosher salt

• 1/4 teaspoon cayenne pepper

Directions

• In a food processor, process all ingredients until smooth.

Apple cinnamon muffins

Ingredients

• 1 cup nonfat plain Greek yogurt

• 2 eggs

• 2 tablespoons canola oil

• 2 teaspoons vanilla extract

• 1 cup all-purpose flour

• 1 cup plus 2 tablespoons sugar

• 3/4 cup milled oats

• 1/4 cup flaxseed meal

• 2 1/4 teaspoons cinnamon

• 1 1/2 teaspoons baking powder

• 1/2 teaspoon salt

• 2 medium peeled and chopped Granny Smith apples

Directions

• Heat oven to 350 F. Lightly coat 2 muffin tins with cooking spray. In a mixing bowl, combine the yogurt, eggs, oil and vanilla. In a medium bowl, combine the flour, 1 cup sugar, oats, flaxseed, 2 teaspoons cinnamon, baking powder and salt. Turn the mixer to low speed. Slowly add the dry ingredients to the wet ingredients. Mix until just combined. Batter should be lumpy. Fold in the apples with a spatula.

• Scoop 1/4 cup of batter into each muffin well. In a small bowl, combine remaining 2 tablespoons sugar and 1/4 teaspoon cinnamon and sprinkle over the batter in each muffin well. Bake for about 22 minutes or until tops are golden brown and toothpick comes out clean when inserted.

Ingredients

• 2 cups all-purpose flour

• 1/2 cup yellow cornmeal

• 1/4 cup packed brown sugar

• 1 tablespoon baking powder

• 1/4 teaspoon salt

• 3/4 cup fat-free milk

• 2 egg whites

• 1 apple, cored, peeled and coarsely chopped

• 1/2 cup corn kernels (fresh or frozen)

Directions

• Heat the oven to 425 F. Line a 12-cup muffin pan with paper or foil liners.

• In a large bowl, combine flour, cornmeal, brown sugar, baking powder and salt. Stir to blend evenly.

• In a separate bowl, combine milk and egg whites. Add chopped apple and corn kernels. Whisk to mix evenly, and pour over the flour mixture. Stir gently until the dry ingredients are slightly moist. The batter will be lumpy.

• Fill prepared muffin cups 2/3 full and bake about 30 minutes. Tops of muffins should spring back to the touch when they're baked.

Best honey whole-wheat bread

Ingredients

• 1 cup dry rolled oats

• 3 cups water

• 3 cups whole-wheat flour

• 3/4 cup soy flour

• 3/4 cup ground flaxseed or flaxseed meal

• 3 tablespoons flaxseed

- 3 tablespoons sesame seeds

- 3 tablespoons poppy seeds

- 4 1/4 tablespoons yeast

- 1 tablespoon sea salt

- 1 cup unsweetened applesauce

- 1/2 cup honey

- 1/4 cup olive oil

- About 5 cups unbleached white flour

Directions

- In microwave-safe bowl, microwave dry rolled oats mixed with water to about 120 F to 130 F. In mixer bowl of a heavy stand mixer with dough hook, combine whole-wheat flour, soy flour, ground flaxseed or flaxseed meal, seeds, yeast, and salt. Stir to mix.

- Add applesauce, honey and oil. Mix by hand. Add the hot rolled oats mixture. Mix by hand.

• When blended, start mixing with dough hook of mixer and continue for about 3 minutes. Slowly add white flour until dough comes away from sides of bowl and becomes smooth and elastic.

• Cover dough in bowl and place in a warm spot. Let rise until about double in size, about 1/2 to 2 hours.

• Punch dough down. Turn onto countertop. Divide evenly into 4 pieces. Shape into 4 loaves. Place in 2 1/2-by-4 1/2-by-8 1/2-inch loaf pans that have been generously sprayed with cooking spray.

• Cover and place in a warm spot. Allow to rise until nearly double in size, about 1 1/2 to 2 hours. Bake at 350 F for 25 minutes, or until tops of loaves are golden. Remove from pans and cool on rack. Cut into half-inch-wide slices.

Carrot and spice quick bread

Ingredients

• 1/2 cup sifted all-purpose flour

• 1 cup whole-wheat flour

• 2 teaspoons baking powder

• 1/2 teaspoon baking soda

• 1/2 teaspoon ground cinnamon

• 1/4 teaspoon ground ginger

• 1/3 cup canola oil

• 1/4 cup, plus 2 tablespoons, firmly packed brown sugar

• 1/3 cup skim milk

• 2 tablespoons unsweetened orange juice

• 2 egg whites, or egg substitute equivalent to 1 egg, beaten

• 1 teaspoon vanilla extract

• 1 teaspoon grated orange rind

• 1 1/2 cups shredded carrots

• 2 tablespoons golden raisins

• 1 tablespoon finely chopped walnuts

Directions

• Heat oven to 375 F. Spray 2 1/2-by-4 1/2-by-8 1/2-inch loaf pan with cooking spray.

• In a small bowl, combine first 6 dry ingredients. Set aside.

• Using a mixer, or stirring vigorously by hand, cream oil and sugar in a large bowl. Beat in milk, orange juice, egg, vanilla and orange rind. Stir in carrots, raisins and walnuts. Add reserved dry ingredients. Mix well.

• Spoon batter into loaf pan. Bake for 45 minutes, or until wooden pick inserted in center comes out clean. Cool in pan 10 minutes. Remove from pan and let cool completely on wire rack.

Cranberry orange muffins

Ingredients

• 8 ounces fat-free plain Greek yogurt

• 2 eggs

• 1/4 cup canola oil

- 1/2 cup granulated sugar

- 1/4 cup brown sugar

- 2 tablespoons unsweetened orange juice concentrate

- 2 tablespoons orange zest

- 2 teaspoons vanilla

- 1 3/4 cup all-purpose flour

- 1/4 cup flaxseed meal

- 1 teaspoon baking powder

- 1 teaspoon baking soda

- 1/8 teaspoon salt

- 1/2 teaspoon cinnamon

- 1 1/2 cups fresh or frozen cranberries

Directions

• Heat the oven to 350 F. Lightly grease muffin tins or place a muffin cup liner in each tin.

• In a mixing bowl, combine the yogurt, eggs, oil, sugars, orange juice concentrate, orange zest and vanilla. In another bowl, combine the flour, flaxseed, baking powder, baking soda, salt and cinnamon. Turn on mixer to low speed and slowly add the dry ingredients to the bowl of wet ingredients. Mix until just incorporated, about 1-2 minutes. Fold in cranberries with a spoon or spatula.

• Scoop 1/4 cup of batter into each muffin well and bake for about 22 minutes or until the tops are golden brown and toothpick comes out clean when inserted.

Irish brown bread

Ingredients

• 2 cups whole-wheat flour

• 1 1/2 cups all-purpose flour, plus extra for kneading and dusting

• 1/2 cup wheat germ

• 2 teaspoons baking soda

• 1/4 teaspoon salt

• 2 cups low-fat buttermilk

• 1 egg, lightly beaten

Directions

• Heat the oven to 400 F. Have ready a nonstick baking sheet.

• In a bowl, combine the flours, wheat germ, baking soda and salt. Whisk to blend. Add buttermilk and egg and stir just until moistened. The dough will be sticky.

• Turn the dough out onto a generously floured work surface and, with floured hands, gently knead it 8 to 10 times. Gather into a loose ball.

• On the baking sheet, form the dough into a 7-inch round. Dust the top of dough with a small amount of flour. Cut a large (4-inch) X into the top of the dough, cutting about 1/2 inch deep.

• Bake until the bread splits open at the X and makes a hollow sound when the underside is tapped, 25 to 30 minutes. Transfer to a wire rack and let cool for 2 hours (ideally) before slicing.

Pumpkin spice muffins

Ingredients

• 2 cups pumpkin puree

• 2 cups nonfat plain Greek yogurt

• 2 eggs

• 1/4 cup canola oil

• 1 teaspoon vanilla extract

• 2 1/2 cups all-purpose flour

• 1 1/2 cups sugar

• 1 1/2 teaspoons cinnamon

• 1 teaspoon baking soda

• 1 teaspoon ground cloves

• 1/4 teaspoon salt

Directions

• Heat the oven to 350 degrees F. Lightly coat 2 muffin tins with cooking spray. In a mixing bowl, combine the pumpkin puree, yogurt, eggs, oil and vanilla. In a medium bowl, combine the flour, sugar, cinnamon, baking soda, cloves and salt. Slowly combine the dry ingredients into the bowl with the wet ingredients, using a mixer. Mix ingredients until just incorporated, about 1 to 2 minutes. Scoop 1/4 cup batter into each muffin well. Bake for 25 to 30 minutes or until muffins spring back when pressed lightly on top and a toothpick comes out clean when inserted.

Three-grain raspberry muffins

Ingredients

• 1/2 cup rolled oats

• 1 cup 1 percent low-fat milk or plain soy milk

• 3/4 cup all-purpose flour

• 1/2 cup cornmeal (preferably coarse-ground)

• 1/4 cup wheat bran

• 1 tablespoon baking powder

• 1/4 teaspoon salt

• 1/2 cup honey

• 3 1/2 tablespoons canola oil

• 2 teaspoons grated lime zest

• 1 egg, lightly beaten

• 2/3 cup raspberries

Directions

• Heat the oven to 400 F. Line a 12-cup muffin pan with paper or foil liners.

• In a large microwave-safe bowl, combine the oats and milk. Microwave on high until the oats are creamy and tender, about 3 minutes. Set aside.

• In a large bowl, combine the flour, cornmeal, bran, baking powder and salt. Whisk to blend. Add the honey, canola oil, lime zest, oat mixture and egg. Beat just until moistened but still slightly lumpy. Gently fold in the raspberries.

• Spoon the batter into the muffin cups, filling each cup about 2/3 full. Bake until the tops are golden brown and a toothpick inserted into the center comes out clean, 16 to 18 minutes. Transfer the muffins to a wire rack and let cool before serving or freezing.

Whole-wheat soda bread

Ingredients

• 2 cups whole-wheat flour

• 1 teaspoon baking powder

• 1/4 cup flaxseed meal (flaxseed flour)

• 1/2 teaspoon baking soda

• 1/4 cup millet meal (millet flour)

• 1 teaspoon caraway seed, crushed

• 2 tablespoons wheat gluten

• 1/4 teaspoon kosher salt

• 1 1/4 cup low-fat buttermilk or skim milk

• 2 egg whites

Directions

• Heat oven to 350 F. In a large bowl, sift together dry ingredients.

• In a separate bowl, combine milk and egg whites. Mix well. Add milk and egg mixture to dry ingredients. Mix until well-moistened.

• Lightly grease the bottom of a 5-by-8-inch loaf pan. Place the dough in the pan. Using a sharp knife, make a slash in the dough lengthwise, about 1/4 inch deep.

• Bake for 50 to 60 minutes. To test for doneness, insert a skewer or knife into the center of the loaf. It should come out clean. Cool thoroughly on a rack before slicing.

Apple-blueberry cobbler

Ingredients

• 2 large apples, peeled, cored and thinly sliced

• 1 tablespoon lemon juice

• 2 tablespoons sugar

• 2 tablespoons cornstarch

• 1 teaspoon ground cinnamon

• 12 ounces fresh or frozen blueberries

For the topping

• 3/4 cup all-purpose flour

• 3/4 cup whole-wheat flour

• 2 tablespoons sugar

• 1 1/2 teaspoons baking powder

• 1/4 teaspoon salt

• 4 tablespoons cold trans-free margarine, cut into pieces

• 1/2 cup fat-free milk

• 1 teaspoon vanilla extract

Directions

• Heat the oven to 400 F. Lightly coat a 9-inch square baking dish with cooking spray.

• In a large bowl, add the apple slices. Sprinkle with lemon juice. In a small bowl, combine the sugar, cornstarch and cinnamon. Add the mixture to the apples and toss gently to mix. Stir in the blueberries. Spread the apple-blueberry mixture evenly in the prepared baking dish. Set aside.

• In another large bowl, combine the flours, sugar, baking powder and salt. Using a fork, cut the cold margarine into the dry ingredients until the mixture resembles coarse crumbs. Add the milk and vanilla. Stir just until a moist dough forms. Turn the dough onto a generously floured work surface and, with floured hands, knead gently 6 to 8 times until the dough is smooth and manageable. Using a rolling pin, roll the dough into a rectangle 1/2-inch thick. Use a cookie cutter to cut out shapes. Cut close together for a minimum of scraps. Gather the scraps and roll out to make more cuts.

• Place the dough pieces over the apple-blueberry mixture until the top is covered. Bake until the apples are tender and the topping is golden, about 30 minutes. Serve warm.

Ingredients

• 1/3 cup dried cherries, coarsely chopped

• 3 tablespoons chopped almonds

• 1 tablespoon wheat germ

• 1 tablespoon firmly packed brown sugar

• 1/2 teaspoon ground cinnamon

• 1/8 teaspoon ground nutmeg

• 6 small Golden Delicious apples, about 1 3/4 pounds total weight

• 1/2 cup apple juice

• 1/4 cup water

• 2 tablespoons dark honey

• 2 teaspoons walnut oil or canola oil

Directions

• Preheat the oven to 350 F.

• In a small bowl, toss together the cherries, almonds, wheat germ, brown sugar, cinnamon and nutmeg until all the ingredients are evenly distributed. Set aside.

• The apples can be left unpeeled, if you like. To peel the apples in a decorative fashion, with a vegetable peeler or a sharp knife, remove the peel from each apple in a circular motion, skipping every other row so that rows of peel alternate with rows of apple flesh. Working from the stem end, core each apple, stopping 3/4 inch from the bottom.

• Divide the cherry mixture evenly among the apples, pressing the mixture gently into each cavity. Arrange the apples upright in a heavy ovenproof frying pan or small baking dish just large enough to hold them. Pour the apple juice and water into the pan. Drizzle the honey and oil evenly over the apples, and cover the pan snugly with aluminum foil. Bake until the apples are tender when pierced with a knife, 50 to 60 minutes.

• Transfer the apples to individual plates and drizzle with the pan juices. Serve warm or at room temperature.

Grilled pineapple

Ingredients

For the marinade

• 2 tablespoons dark honey

• 1 tablespoon olive oil

• 1 tablespoon fresh lime juice

• 1 teaspoon ground cinnamon

• 1/4 teaspoon ground cloves

• 1 firm, ripe pineapple

• 8 wooden skewers, soaked in water for 30 minutes, or metal skewers

• 1 tablespoon dark rum (optional)

• 1 tablespoon grated lime zest

Directions

• Prepare a hot fire in a charcoal grill or heat a gas grill or broiler. Away from the heat source, lightly coat the grill rack or broiler pan with cooking spray. Position the cooking rack 4 to 6 inches from the heat source.

• To make the marinade, in a small bowl, combine the honey, olive oil, lime juice, cinnamon and cloves and whisk to blend. Set aside.

• Cut off the crown of leaves and the base of the pineapple. Stand the pineapple upright and, using a large, sharp knife, pare off the skin, cutting downward just below the surface in long, vertical strips and leaving the small brown "eyes" on the fruit.

• Lay the pineapple on its side. Aligning the knife blade with the diagonal rows of eyes, cut a shallow furrow, following a spiral pattern around the pineapple, to remove all the eyes.

• Stand the peeled pineapple upright and cut it in half lengthwise. Place each pineapple half cut-side down and cut it lengthwise into four long wedges. Slice away the core. Cut each wedge crosswise into three pieces. Thread the three pineapple pieces onto each skewer.

• Lightly brush the pineapple with the marinade. Grill or broil, turning once and basting once or twice with the remaining marinade, until tender and golden, about 5 minutes on each side.

• Remove the pineapple from the skewers and place on a platter or individual serving plates. Brush with the rum, if using, and sprinkle with the lime zest. Serve hot or warm.

Mixed berry whole-grain coffeecake

Ingredients

• 1/2 cup skim milk

• 1 tablespoon vinegar

• 2 tablespoons canola oil

• 1 teaspoon vanilla

• 1 egg

• 1/3 cup packed brown sugar

• 1 cup whole-wheat pastry flour

• 1/2 teaspoon baking soda

• 1/2 teaspoon ground cinnamon

• 1/8 teaspoon salt

• 1 cup frozen mixed berries, such as blueberries, raspberries and blackberries (do not thaw)

• 1/4 cup low-fat granola, slightly crushed

Directions

• Heat oven to 350 F. Spray an 8-inch round cake pan with cooking spray and coat with flour.

• In a large bowl, mix the milk, vinegar, oil, vanilla, egg and brown sugar until smooth. Stir in flour, baking soda, cinnamon and salt just until moistened. Gently fold half the berries into the batter. Spoon into the prepared pan. Sprinkle with remaining berries and top with the granola.

• Bake 25 to 30 minutes or until golden brown and top springs back when touched in center. Cool in pan on cooling rack for 10 minutes. Serve warm.

Beef and vegetable kebabs

Ingredients

• 1/2 cup brown rice

• 2 cups water

• 4 ounces top sirloin (choice)

• 1 tablespoon fat-free Italian dressing

• 1 green pepper, seeded and cut into 4 pieces

• 4 cherry tomatoes

• 1 small onion, cut into 4 wedges

• 2 wooden skewers, soaked in water for 30 minutes, or metal skewers

Directions

• In a saucepan over high heat, combine the rice and water. Bring to a boil. Reduce the heat to low, cover and simmer until the water is absorbed and the rice is tender, about 30 to 45 minutes. Add more water if necessary to keep the rice from drying out. Transfer to a small bowl to keep warm.

• Cut the meat into 4 equal portions. Put the meat in a small bowl and pour Italian dressing over the top. Rub the dressing into each piece. Cover and place in the refrigerator for at least 20 minutes to marinate, turning as needed.

• Prepare a hot fire in a charcoal grill or heat a gas grill or a broiler. Away from the heat source, lightly coat the grill rack or broiler pan with cooking spray. Position the cooking rack 4 to 6 inches from the heat source.

• Thread 2 cubes of meat, 2 green pepper pieces, 2 cherry tomatoes and 2 onion wedges onto each skewer. Place the kebabs on the grill rack or broiler pan. Grill or broil the kebabs for about 5 to 10 minutes, turning as needed.

• Divide the rice onto individual plates. Top with 1 kebab and serve immediately.

Broccoli, garlic and rigatoni

Ingredients

• 1/3 pound whole-wheat rigatoni

• 2 cups broccoli florets (tops)

• 2 tablespoons Parmesan cheese

• 2 teaspoons olive oil

• 2 teaspoons minced garlic

• Freshly ground black pepper, to taste

Directions

• Fill a large pot 3/4 full with water and bring to a boil. Add the pasta and cook until al dente (tender), 10 to 12 minutes, or according to the package directions. Drain the pasta thoroughly.

• While the pasta is cooking, in a pot fitted with a steamer basket, bring 1 inch of water to a boil. Add the broccoli, cover and steam until tender, about 10 minutes.

• In a large bowl, combine the cooked pasta and broccoli. Toss with Parmesan cheese, olive oil and garlic. Season with pepper to taste. Serve immediately.

Apple Almond Galette

Ingredients

• 4 baking apples, peeled, cored and sliced thin

• 1 tablespoon butter

• 2 teaspoons ground cinnamon

• ⅛ teaspoon ground ginger

• 2 tablespoons brown sugar

• 9 individual Stevia packets

• 2 teaspoons almond extract

• 1 store-bought 9" layer pie crust

Directions

• Over medium low heat, cook butter, apples, cinnamon, ginger and brown sugar for 5 to 10 minutes; until the apples become soft.

• Turn off the heat and stir in the Stevia and the almond extract.

• Pre–heat your oven to 400 F.

• Roll out the pie crust onto a cookie sheet.

• Pour the apple mixture into the middle of the pie crust.

• Fold the pie crust over the apples about 3", leaving the center uncovered.

• Pinch the creases together and bake for 30 minutes or until the pie crust is golden brown.

Ingredients

• 5 Granny Smith Apples, peeled, cored and sliced

• ¼ cup lemon juice

• ¼ cup Caramel Flavoring, sugar free

• ⅓ cup All Purpose (AP) flour

• ¼ cup butter

• 1 cup Oatmeal

• 2 Tablespoons cinnamon

• Butter spray

Directions

• Toss sliced apples in lemon juice; pour off any extra lemon juice.

• Soak apple slices in caramel flavoring for 10 minutes.

• Pre-heat oven to 375 degrees Fahrenheit.

• Lightly oil an 8X8 pan, place apples in the bottom.

• In a bowl mix flour, oatmeal and cinnamon together; then cut in the butter, until you have small pieces, sprinkle the mixture over the top of the apples.

• Bake for 40 minutes; spray the top with a butter spray and bake for another 5 minutes.

Apple Cranberry Walnut Salad

Ingredients

• 2 cups Red Seedless Grapes, each grape sliced in half

• 1⅓ cups Walnut Halves, chopped into small pea-size pieces

• 1¼ cups Pomegranate Infused Ocean Spray Dried Cranberries, 1-6-ounce package

• 4 stalks Celery, chopped into quarter-inch pieces

• 7 hmedium-sized Gala Apples skin on

• 8 fluid ounce bottle of Maple Grove Farms of Vermont Fat-Free Cranberry Balsamic Dressing

Directions

• Rinse cluster of red grapes and separate from the stem. Use paring knife and slice each grape in half. Place sliced grapes in extra large mixing bowl.

• Measure walnut halves into measuring cup. Can use a nut chopper to chop nuts into pea size pieces or put walnuts in a plastic sandwich baggie, seal and use the bottom of the 1 cup measure to gently press on the walnuts to break the walnuts into pea size like pieces. Add chopped nuts to the extra large mixing bowl with the slice red grapes.

• Add one 6 ounce bag of dried pomegranate infused cranberries to the grape and walnut mixture.

• Rinse, clean and chop celery in quarter inch pieces, add to the grape, walnut, and dried cranberry mixture.

• Rinse the seven Gala apples, slice in half vertically and core the apples. Make 5 apple wedges and then slice the wedges into bite size, quarter in pieces. Add chopped apple pieces to the rest of the mixture.

• Pour the 8 fluid ounce bottle of cranberry dressing over the entire mixture. Stir the ingredients making sure that the dressing is incorporated and covers all of the ingredients. Chill and serve.

Apple Sage Stuffing

Ingredients

• 1 teaspoon Canola oil

• 1 large yellow onion, diced

• 4 stalks of celery, diced

• 2 Granny Smith apples, peeled, cored and diced

• 2 tablespoons ground sage

• 1 tablespoon poultry spice

• 1½ cups apple cider

• 1 cup low–sodium chicken stock

• 12 cups of cubed low–sodium bread (¾ to 1 whole loaf)

Directions

• In a large fry pan, add oil, onions, celery and apples and sauté until onions are translucent.

• Add sage, poultry spice, apple cider and chicken stock; simmer for 10 minutes.

• Place cubed bread on a cooking sheet and bake in a pre-heated 400F oven until the bread is brown, turning the cubes occasional to brown all sides.

• When bread cubes are brown add to the fry pan and mix together.

• Bake the dressing in a covered 9 X 13 pan in a 350° F oven for 20 to 30 minutes.

Apple Spice Cake

Ingredients

• 3 Granny Smith Apples, peeled, cored & sliced

• 1 yellow sugar-free cake mix

• 3 egg whites

• ½ cup water

• ⅓ cup oil

• 1 teaspoon ground nutmeg

• 1 teaspoon ground ginger

• 1 teaspoon ground cinnamon

• ½ teaspoon ground cloves

• 3 tablespoons maple sugar

Directions

• Microwave apple slices until soft, about 5 minutes on high.

• Pre-heat the oven to 350.

• Let the apple cool, while you mix the cake batter.

• In a mixing bowl, add the cake mix, spices, egg whites, water and oil; follow the mixing direction on the box.

• Mix in the apples.

• Pour the batter into a non-stick 9 X 13 cake pan.

• Bake until the cake is done (a tooth pick comes out clean), 35 to 45 minutes. (Remember, there is very little sugar in this batter, so the cake doesn't brown.)

• Let cool to room temperature.

• Sprinkle the top of the cake with maple sugar.

Ingredients

• 1 lb. asparagus

• 1 oz. dried wild mushroom medley

• 1 cup very hot water

• 2 teaspoon olive oil

• 2 celery stalks

• 1 carrot stick

- 1 small onion

- 1 fennel (anise) head

- 4 sprigs fresh thyme

- pinch cayenne pepper

- ground black pepper to taste

- 1 teaspoon dried sage

- 1 tablespoon fresh chopped parsley

- 1 tablespoon + 1 teaspoon dry Marsala wine

- 1 bay leaf

- ⅛ teaspoon garlic powder

- ⅛ teaspoon onion powder

- 2 cups vegetable stock, low sodium

- 2 oz. pine nuts

Directions

• Preheat oven to 400° F. Wash and cut off the tough bottoms of asparagus spears.

• Place the asparagus spears into a single layer on a baking sheet. Spray the spears with olive oil. (1 teaspoon olive oil sprayed on spears) Bake in the oven for 10 minutes. Allow the spears to cool and cut into 1-inch pieces.

• Reconstitute dried mushrooms in 1 cup very hot water.

• Heat 1 teaspoon olive oil in non-stick sauce pan over medium-high heat and add diced celery, carrots, onions, and fennel and saut until onions are translucent. Add thyme, cayenne pepper, sage, chopped parsley, Marsala wine, bay leaf, garlic powder, onion powder, and keep stirring for 1 more minute over heat. Add vegetable stock, liquid from the dried mushrooms, diced wild mushrooms, and simmer for 15 minutes.

• Place the asparagus pieces in the bottom of the dish, add stew and sprinkle pine nuts over the top and serve.

Baked Salmon with Roasted Asparagus on Cracked Wheat Bun

Ingredients

- 16 oz. fresh salmon fillet

- 1 tablespoon lemon juice

- 1 tablespoon butter

- 12 oz. fresh asparagus spears (woody stems removed), washed

- 1 tablespoon olive oil

- 4 cracked wheat or whole-grain hamburger buns, toasted

Directions

- Preheat oven to 400°F.

- Place asparagus spears on a cookie sheet and spray with olive oil.

- Roast in the oven for 10 minutes or until tender and slightly brown.

- Remove from the oven and allow to cool.

Ingredients

• 12 button mushrooms, stems removed

• ¼ cup balsamic vinegar

• ¼ cup apple cider vinegar

• 1 tbsp. chopped chive + extra for garnish

• Pinch freshly ground black pepper

Directions

• In a medium sized bowl or Tupperware, place the mushrooms with the rest of the ingredients and cover.

• Use hands to mix everything together and then place in the refrigerator for a minimum of 2 hours and a maximum of 2 days, shaking every so often to redistribute the vinegar dressing.

• To serve, take the mushrooms out of the bowl or Tupperware, separate them from the vinegar, and sprinkle with extra chives. You can also add an extra drizzle of the leftover vinegar on top of the mushrooms. Or get even fancier by reducing the vinegar (by placing in a pot, on the stove, and cooking over medium heat) and using it as a thicker sauce.

BBQ Apple Chips

Ingredients

• 1 apple (Granny Smith, Golden Delicious, or Fuji)

• Parchment paper

• 1 tbsp smoked paprika

• 2 tsp chili powder

• 2 tsp cumin

• 1 tsp salt-free onion powder

• 1 tsp salt-free garlic powder

• 1 tsp brown sugar

• 1 tsp freshly cracked black pepper

• ¼ tsp mustard powder

Directions

• Preheat oven to 225 degrees F.

• Core your apple and then, using a mandoline, cut it into 1/8-inch slices. Time-saver tip: If you don't want to core the apple, you can pull out the seeds with your fingers after slicing. And if you don't have a mandoline, you can make thin slices with your knife.

• Next, cover two 9x11-inch baking sheets with parchment paper and set aside.

• In a small bowl, mix the spice ingredients together.

• Place a few apple slices on a large plate and rub the spice mix on both sides.

• Set slices in a single layer on the parchment-lined baking sheet.

• Continue until all the apple slices are spiced and placed on the sheet. Place the apples in the oven and bake for one hour. Flip the slices over and bake for another hour.

• Then, turn the oven off but leave the apples inside to cool - this is when they get nice and crispy.

• Serve and enjoy immediately or keep in an airtight container for a few days.

BBQ Pineapple Chicken

Ingredients

• 4 oz skinless chicken breast, diced into 2-inch cubes

• 20 oz can pineapple rings

• 2 tsp chopped garlic

• 1 tsp dijon mustard

• ½ tsp wasabi paste

Directions

• Remove pineapple rings from can and save the drained pineapple juice.

• Mix pineapple juice with garlic, mustard and wasibi paste.

• Dice chicken breasts into 2 inch cubes.

• Combine Pineapple juice mixture and chicken together and marinate over night in the refrigerator.

• Place the chicken pieces on skewers or grill on the barbeque on a metal grate.

• Barbecue chicken on a hot grill until the chicken is golden brown and is cooked in the center (5 to 10 minutes depending upon the temperature of your grill)

Very Berry Tofu Smoothie

Ingredients

• 1 lb fresh strawberries, cleaned and hulled

• 2 cups blueberries

• 9 oz tofu, silken, extra firm

• ½ teaspoon ground ginger

• 2 pinches of red pepper flakes

- ¼ teaspoon rum extract

- 1 tablespoon honey

- 1 teaspoon lemon juice

- ½ cup ice

Directions

- Blend all together and serve.

Blueberry Lemon Pound Cake

Ingredients

- ½ cup non-fat cottage cheese

- ½ cup unsalted butter

- 3 fresh eggs

- 1 cup fat-free lemon yogurt

- 2 tsp vanilla extract

- ¼ cup Splenda

• 1¼ cup all-purpose flour

• ½ cup whole wheat flour

• 1 tsp baking powder

• ½ tsp baking soda

• ¼ tsp salt

• 2 tsp lemon zest

• 1 cup blueberries

Directions

• Puree cottage cheese till smooth.

• Place cottage cheese puree, butter, Splenda in a mixer and beat till smooth.

• Add eggs, yogurt, vanilla, lemon juice, lemon zest, and blend until smooth.

• Scrape sides of the bowl. Sift dry ingredients, all-purpose flour, whole wheat flour, baking powder, baking soda, and salt.

• Add to mixing bowl, blend until smooth.

• Add blueberries and mix them into the rest of the batter.

• Pour mixture into greased 8" angel food cake pan.

• Bake for 35-40 minutes at 375°F.

Ingredients

• 5½ oz of ground beef or turkey

• 2 medium onions, chopped in cubes

• 1 medium eggplant, peeled and cut in cubes

• 4 cloves of garlic, chopped

• 1 medium carrot, peeled and grated or chopped finely

• 1 small red pepper, seeded and chopped

• 2 Tbsp tomato paste (low salt)

• ¼ tsp black pepper

• 2 Tbsp canola oil

• 4 cups water

• 4 tsp cornstarch for thickening

• 2 Tbsp olive oil

• 10 oz Rice noodles

Directions

• In a deep skillet, sauté onions in oil until soft.

• Add the beef and brown for 1-2 minutes while stirring.

• Add the eggplant and continue to stir for an additional 1-2 minutes.

• Add the remainder of the ingredients, except for the cornstarch and olive oil.

• Bring to a boil, lower the fire and cook covered on medium flame for 20 minutes, stirring occasionally and checking that it is not burning.

• Mix the cornstarch in 1/4 cup of cold water, add to the skillet while stirring.

• Bring to a boil again for 1/2 a minute and remove from the fire.

• Rice Noodles

• Soak the noodles in a large amount of boiling water, take off the heat for 10 minutes, or cook in boiling water for 2 minutes.

• Rinse and mix with sauce mixture.

• Add the olive oil, mix and serve.

Bow-Tie Pasta Salad

Ingredients

• 2 cups cooked bow-tie pasta

• ¼ cup chopped celery

• 2 tablespoons chopped green pepper

• 2 tablespoons shredded carrot

• 2 tablespoons minced onion

• ⅛ teaspoon pepper

• ⅔ cup mayonnaise, low-fat

• ½ teaspoon sugar

• 1 tablespoon lemon juice

Directions

• Mix pasta, celery, green pepper, carrot and onion in a bowl.

• In separate small bowl, blend pepper, mayonnaise, sugar and lemon juice until smooth.

• Pour over pasta and vegetables.

• Mix until well coated.

• Chill before serving.

www.ingramcontent.com/pod-product-compliance
Lightning Source LLC
Chambersburg PA
CBHW070816170726
48000CB00017B/929